YOUR KNOWLEDGE HAS VALUE

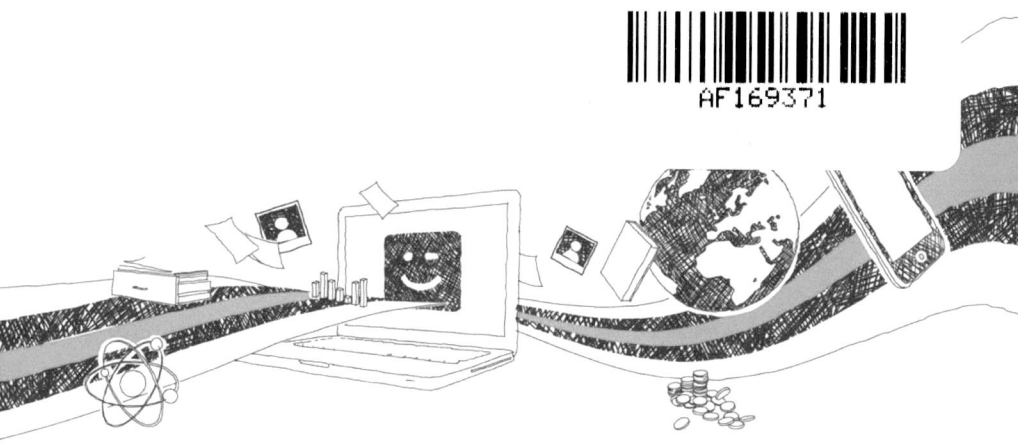

- We will publish your bachelor's and master's thesis, essays and papers

- Your own eBook and book - sold worldwide in all relevant shops

- Earn money with each sale

Upload your text at www.GRIN.com
and publish for free

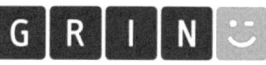

Bibliographic information published by the German National Library:

The German National Library lists this publication in the National Bibliography; detailed bibliographic data are available on the Internet at http://dnb.dnb.de .

This book is copyright material and must not be copied, reproduced, transferred, distributed, leased, licensed or publicly performed or used in any way except as specifically permitted in writing by the publishers, as allowed under the terms and conditions under which it was purchased or as strictly permitted by applicable copyright law. Any unauthorized distribution or use of this text may be a direct infringement of the author s and publisher s rights and those responsible may be liable in law accordingly.

Imprint:

Copyright © 2018 GRIN Verlag
Print and binding: Books on Demand GmbH, Norderstedt Germany
ISBN: 9783668626331

This book at GRIN:

https://www.grin.com/document/388520

Patrick Kimuyu

Treatment and Nursing Management of Tuberculosis

GRIN Verlag

GRIN - Your knowledge has value

Since its foundation in 1998, GRIN has specialized in publishing academic texts by students, college teachers and other academics as e-book and printed book. The website www.grin.com is an ideal platform for presenting term papers, final papers, scientific essays, dissertations and specialist books.

Visit us on the internet:

http://www.grin.com/

http://www.facebook.com/grincom

http://www.twitter.com/grin_com

Treatment and Nursing Management of Tuberculosis

Name: Patrick Kimuyu

Inhaltsverzeichnis

Introduction 3
    Elements in the chain of infection of tuberculosis 3
    Reservoir: 3
    Portal of Exit: 4
    Means of Transmission: 4
    Portal of Entry: 5
    Susceptible Host: 5
Nursing Management of Tuberculosis 6
    Treatment Options 6
    Role of Professional Nurses in TB management 7
    Evidence-based Practice Nursing Intervention 8
References 10

Introduction

In practice, evidence-based practice helps in developing appropriate control and prevention measures of infectious diseases. However, effective intervention relies on an informed understanding of the chain of infection. This is a paramount aspect in professional nursing because it facilitates nursing management of a given condition with the focus of breaking the chain through treatment and nursing management interventions.

Elements in the chain of infection of tuberculosis

In the case of tuberculosis, the chain of infection involves six key elements. These elements are infectious agent, reservoir, portal of exit, means of transmission, portal of entry, and susceptible host.

Infectious agent: Etiological agent of tuberculosis in humans has been found to be a bacterium known as *Mycobaterium tuberculosis*. *M. tuberculosis* is a pathogenic bacterium, and it belongs to Mycobacteriaceae family. This bacterium exhibits unique microbiological characteristics which are responsible for its pathogenicity. *M. tuberculosis* is a nonmotile bacterium which thrives in environments with high oxygen levels. As such, it is considered as an obligate aerobe. From the bacteriological staining, *M. tuberculosis* is considered as an acid-fast bacterium. It possesses a complex cellwall which comprises of mycolic acids, a characteristic that confer it with resistance to weak disinfectants. Genetic studies indicate that *M. tuberculosis* consists of 167 strains which are responsible for 98.8% of tuberculosis cases in humans (Assam et al., 2013).

Reservoir:

Reservoir for *M. tuberculosis* is another human being in which the bacterium thrives. Ordinarily, M. tuberculosis thrives in natural environments with high levels of oxygen. This is why it prefers the mammalian respiratory tract. However, it is worth noting that *M. tuberculosis* can infect different regions of the body. Apart from the respiratory tract, especially the lungs, this bacterium infects the spine where it may cause lifelong disability.

Portal of Exit:

Portal of exit for *M. tuberculosis* is through cough or sneeze through which the etiological agent is propelled into air (World Health Organization, 2015). Biological analysis indicates that sputum contains a high population of the bacilli. This is why diagnosis for tuberculosis involves sputum analysis including acid-fast staining and microscopy to identify the stained rods. In addition, bacterial culture techniques are useful in which sputum is cultured to determine growth of the rods. Therefore, propulsion of sputum into the air through coughing, spitting or sneezing serves as the portal of exit for tuberculosis.

Means of Transmission:

Tuberculosis is known as an airborne disease because its transmission occurs through the air. Ordinarily, the route of transmission of tuberculosis is direct from the reservoir person to the new susceptible individual or host. Transmission occurs when a person with tuberculosis propels respiratory droplets into the air through coughing or sneezing. In most cases, these are microscopic droplets that can be propelled through singing, laughing and speaking. However, it is worth noting that only persons with active tuberculosis can spread the bacteria (National Institutes of Health, 2012). According to World Health Organization (2015), tuberculosis in humans can exist in active or latent forms. It is reported that one-third of the global population is infected with latent tuberculosis. These persons cannot transmit tuberculosis to other people. This implies that only persons with active tuberculosis can spread it directly to other people, especially those in damp and overcrowded environments which are characterized by limited space such as small houses (Müller, 2011).

On the other hand, transmission of tuberculosis can occur when dust contaminated with TB bacilli enter into the body of uninfected person. As such, dusty environments favor the spread of tuberculosis (Müller, 2011).

Portal of Entry:

Infection of tuberculosis occurs when uninfected person inhales respiratory droplets which are propelled by a person suffering from tuberculosis into air. Therefore, inhalation serves as the portal of entry into the body. Upon entry into the body, tuberculosis bacilli infect the respiratory tract, primarily the lungs where they multiply and exert their pathology. However, it is worth noting that tuberculosis cannot be transmitted from a pregnant mother to the fetus because tuberculosis bacilli do not cross the placenta (Müller, 2011).

Susceptible Host:

Humans serve as the hosts for tuberculosis. M. tuberculosis can infect all people irrespective of gender, race and color. As such, the disease does not exhibit demographic inequalities. However, tuberculosis exists in people in two distinct forms: inactive and active. People with latent tuberculosis do not exhibit the pathology related to the disease. However, latent tuberculosis can become active and this is manifested by the main signs and symptoms of tuberculosis.

World Health Organization (2015) reports that, people with latent tuberculosis have a 10% risk of developing active tuberculosis. This risk is related to several factors which increase an individual's susceptibility to tuberculosis. First, people with suppressed immune system are highly susceptible to tuberculosis infection. For instance, HIV patients are highly susceptible to tuberculosis in a situation referred to as co-infection. Babies are also more susceptible to tuberculosis infection than healthy adults. Second, malnutrition increases the risk of getting tuberculosis infection. Moreover, smoking increases an individual's susceptibility to tuberculosis.

Nursing Management of Tuberculosis

Treatment Options

In practice, treatment of tuberculosis focuses on destroying the etiological agents through the use of therapeutic agents, primarily antibiotics. The chain of infection of tuberculosis is broken through administering appropriate regiments to an infected person. On the other hand, preventive measures such as vaccination can protect susceptible individuals especially children from acquiring tuberculosis. Despite the risk posed by tuberculosis, appropriate treatment and nursing management reduces deaths associated to the disease. However, it is worth noting that treatment options depend on the nature of infection.

In pulmonary tuberculosis, the patient is put on anti-infective agents referred to as primary drugs. This treatment regime comprises of a combination of two drugs: isoniazid and rifampin or ethambutol. This is usually a short-course therapy that lasts for 6 months. On the other hand, pyrazinamide and streptomycin or ethambutol are administered to a patient for a minimum of 2 months after which isoniazid therapy is initiated for 3 more moths. In case isoniazid resistance is suspected, ethambutol combined with pyrazinamide, streptomycin or rifapentine are administered to a tuberculosis patient for two months.

Second-line drugs are used for extended therapy that may be continued for up to 24 months. Drugs used for extended therapy include ethionamide, capreomycin and para-aminosalicylate. This treatment option is indicated for patients with long-term consequences of tuberculosis infection. For instance, reactivated tuberculosis and other medical problems such as silicosis or diabetes mellitus require patients to be put on second-line drugs.

In a patient with extrapulmonary tuberculosis, primary drugs; isoniazid and rifampin are administered to the patient for 6 months. However, a patient with extrapulmonary tuberculosis that affects the brain may require prescription with corticosteroids, primarily prednisolone to be taken together with anti-TB drugs. This is usually necessary in reducing inflammation in the affected areas (NHS, 2014).

Latent TB is treated with a combination of isoniazid and rifampin for 3 months. Alternatively, latent TB can be treated through the administration of isoniazid alone for 6 months. However, it is worth noting that treatment of latent TB is not recommended to all patients. For instance, this treatment is recommended to healthcare workers, HIV patients and people with tuberculosis-caused scarring. In addition, this treatment option is not recommended to patients with latent TB aged beyond 35 years. Moreover, patients who are on chemotherapy, long-term corticosteroids or tumor-necrosis factor inhibitors require treatment for latent TB because these medical interventions increase the risk of latent TB activation (NHS, 2014).

Role of Professional Nurses in TB management

It is apparent that professional nurses play pivotal roles infection control and prevention of tuberculosis, as well as in other diseases. In tuberculosis management, several aspects of treatment are supposed to be considered, in order to break the infection. One of the most principal management aspects is adherence to treatment. Over the past few decades, drug resistance has been identified to a significant barrier to effective treatment. Treatment of tuberculosis with one drug regimen for long periods has been found to lead to the development multi-drug resistant (MDR) tuberculosis strains (Bernstein, 2015). These M. tuberculosis variants are difficult to treat; thus they cause devastating consequences. Therefore, professional nurses are essential in controlling tuberculosis infection because they facilitate appropriate identification and prevention of new TB cases. More importantly, nurses ensure timely start of TB treatment, as well as providing the necessary support to patients during treatment (Murphy, 2015).

Evidence-based Practice Nursing Intervention

The first nursing intervention is reviewing the pathology of tuberculosis, in order to gain an overview of TB progression and spread of infection. The rationale for this intervention is to facilitate adherence to TB treatment by the patient. The patient is able to understand the importance of adhering to treatment, in order to prevent complications associated to TB management including drug-resistance or reactivation (Vera, 2013). In addition, this intervention will help the patient adopt appropriate measures to prevent the spread of TB to other people after gaining knowledge on transmission.

The second nursing intervention is to identify other people who may be exposed to the risk of TB infection. For instance, this process can involve family members and friends or close associates. The rationale for this intervention is to prevent the spread of infection, especially to household members.

Third, a review of proper waste disposal and hygiene is necessary to prevent behaviors that promote the spread of tuberculosis. For instance, the patient can be instructed to follow high hygienic standards such as hand washing, and observing caution when sneezing, coughing, or even laughing. The patient should be taught on how to cough expectorate into a tissue for disposal. In addition, the patient should be instructed to refrain from spitting, in order to prevent the spread of TB infection (Vera, 2013).

On the other hand, the nurse should evaluate the level of patient's cooperation to ensure uninterrupted drug therapy. The patient should be informed of the significance of drug compliance. The rationale for this intervention is to prevent infection during the contagious period, usually up to 3 months following chemotherapy initiation. In cases of long-term treatment with multidrug regimens, directly-observed therapy is necessary to enhance compliance.

Moreover, the nurse should review the significance of periodic reculturing of sputum and follow-up check-ups during treatment therapy. The rationale for this intervention is to identify any possible resistance to primary drugs that may warrant the extension of therapy second-line drugs up to 24 months. Finally, the nurse should encourage or provide well-balanced meals to the patient, in order to promote the functioning of the immune system (Vera, 2013).

References

Assam, J. P., et al. (2013). Mycobacterium Tuberculosis Is The Causative Agent Of Tuberculosis In The Southern Ecological Zones Of Cameroon, As Shown By Genetic Analysis. *BMC Infectious Diseases*, 13:431.

Bernstein, L. B. (2015). *Understanding Tuberculosis - Diagnosis and Treatment*. Retrieved from http://www.webmd.com/a-to-z-guides/understanding-tuberculosis-treatment?page=2

Müller, A. (2011). *How TB is Spread*. Retrieved from http://www.tbonline.info/posts/2011/5/27/how-tb-spread/

National Institutes of Health (2012). *Tuberculosis*. Retrieved from http://www.niaid.nih.gov/topics/tuberculosis/understanding/pages/transmission.aspx

NHS (2014). *Tuberculosis (TB) – Treatment*. Retrieved from http://www.nhs.uk/Conditions/Tuberculosis/Pages/Treatment.aspx

Vera, M. (2013). *5 Pulmonary Tuberculosis Nursing Care Plans*. Retrieved from http://nurseslabs.com/5-pulmonary-tuberculosis-nursing-care-plans/

World Health Organization (2015). *What Is TB? How Is It Treated?* Retrieved from http://www.who.int/features/qa/08/en/

YOUR KNOWLEDGE HAS VALUE

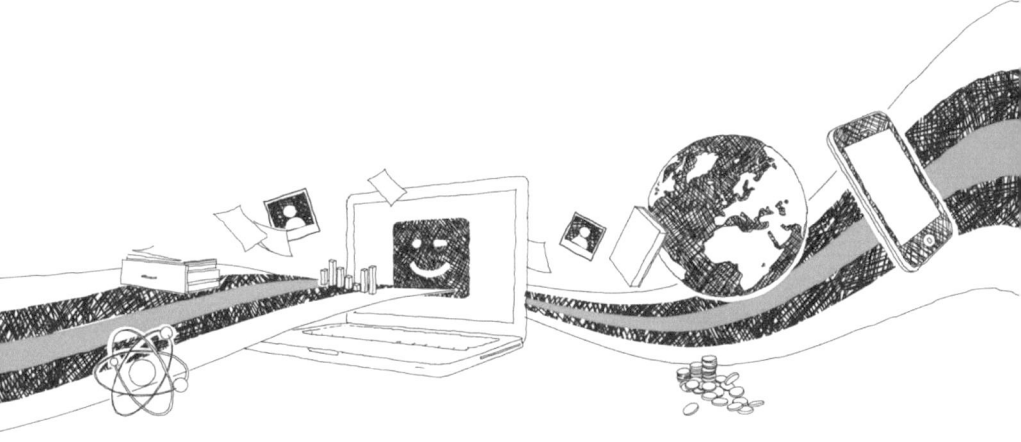

- We will publish your bachelor's and master's thesis, essays and papers

- Your own eBook and book - sold worldwide in all relevant shops

- Earn money with each sale

Upload your text at www.GRIN.com
and publish for free

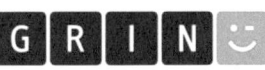